AF885043

Youth Rise:

Substance Abuse Treatment Program

A Poly-Therapeutic Substance Abuse Treatment Manual for Providers

Written by Justin Nutt, LSCSW, LCSW

Product of Nurstead Consulting Services

How to Use This Manual

The information in this manual is intended to allow qualified mental health professionals and domestic violence workers to deliver group cognitive behavioral and dialectical behavioral treatment for individuals who have developed a pattern of unhealthy and/or abusive relationships. Each of the twelve 90-120 minute sessions are divided into five sections:

- **Instructions to Group Leaders**
- **Check In Procedure** (to start with second session)
- **Suggested Remarks**
- **Worksheet**
- **Worksheet Review**

The Instructions to Group Leaders section summarizes what information is to be presented in the session and outlines key components of the session. The Check In Procedure section provides a process by which members check in each session as a way of building trust and relationships within the group. The Suggested Remarks section provides a narrative which allows for the group leader to provide the information that is to be covered in that session. ***While it is not necessary to recite the script verbatim the group leader should deliver the information as closely as possible to the way which it is in the script.*** It is suggested that group leaders also include events connected to the topic in their presentation to help participants see how the concepts would play out in real life. After the presentation of information, the group members should be given time to complete the worksheet connected to the topic and then the worksheet questions should be asked as a review of what was learned in the session. The Worksheet Review section allows for a discussion of the worksheet each participant completed during the session. Each participant will report on his or her own worksheet, and then others members are invited to discuss the participant's report.

Group leaders need to monitor time, and on occasion limit responses and discussion from each member, so that all necessary information can be provided within the 90 minutes that each session is to last. Limitation of some group members may be needed so that other members are allowed time to discuss their worksheet and feel connected to the assignment and discussion topic. The need for limiting will be in direct connection to the number of members included in the group. Larger groups or more intense topics or discussions may create the need for the session to last the full 90 minutes, and smaller groups and topics may allow for sessions to be completed in 60 minutes.

Check In:

Check in may vary depending upon the setting and clients enrolled. In addition to what is listed as the recommended check in topic there are additional items which can be used as part of check in to assist in the therapeutic process.

Emotion Based Check In:

When using the emotion based check in process, an additional question the group leader should have each member of the group answer is "*Are you mad, glad, sad, or afraid?*" Once the person has identified the feeling and stated what made him/her choose that emotion, emotional awareness may occur. If a group member chooses glad, the perspective of looking for positives should be reinforced. If the person chooses sad or mad, these items should be explored, and questions should be asked which assist the person in discovering any underlying emotions. So long as the group member is able to answer the questions, each layer of emotion should be peeled back until the base emotion is discovered.

Positive and Negative Check In:

This method is used to assist group participants in gaining awareness of positive events and acceptance of negative events. In addition to the suggested check in questions, when using the positive and negative check in method, you will also want to have each group member state a positive and a negative event (mountains and valleys) which has occurred since the last group session. Some group members may consistently look at only the positive or negative in life, and this check in technique is designed to help these members to not focus on only one aspect of a situation, but to also understand that there is positive, negative, and in between in all aspects of life.

Check Outs:

Just as the check in process helps group members enter a learning mindset which promotes engagement during the group session, check outs can assist with members exiting the group session and help them prepare to learn the safety of a therapeutic intervention and to face life. The most common check out question is to ask what each member learned from the session, but check out is commonly used when there is a holiday approaching which may have the ability to impact the group members and hinder sobriety. If this is the case, the suggested check out question is that of *"What are your plans for the holiday?"* and "*How can you protect your sobriety over the holiday?*" A check in helps to define the start of a session and allows members to settle and engage, and as such, it is a needed aspect of the therapeutic approach, but a check out is something which may or may not be used.

Cognitive Distortions

SESSION 1:

Instructions to Group Leaders:

The purpose of the first session is to develop group rules with help of participants, work to lay foundations of trust between group members, and to discuss the format which subsequent session will follow. This session will also cover cognitive distortions. The portions related to group norms can be removed if this is an open and revolving group instead of a closed group with members all starting at the same time.

Suggested Remarks:

Introductions and Group Rules:

1. Each session we will use a round robin process to start the session. This process helps us to break the ice, but also to learn more about each of the other participants in the group.

2. To start this session, since you may or may not know others in the group, I would like each of you to introduce yourself and also tells us your favorite food.

3. Since an important part of the group process for healing to occur is openness, there is the need for some group rules to be established.
    a. Group safety: No violence or threats towards staff or other group members is allowed.
    b. Confidentiality: It is important that whatever is said in the group is kept within the group. Just as you would not want for other members to tell what you have shared outside the group, other members also do not want for their information to be shared outside the group.
    c. Respect: It is important that each member of the group be respected and while you may not agree with another member's beliefs, they are still worthy of respect, just as you are. This doesn't mean that in discussions you cannot state an opposing viewpoint; challenging of beliefs with respect to relationships is an integral part of the group process as other members may see things in a way the person cannot, but when doing so it is expected that you will be respectful. Respect also means that you will not cut another group member off, but let him or her finish before you speak.
    d. Participation: Some members may be more comfortable sharing than others, but for the group process to work, all participants need to participate. Along with this it is also

important to let other people talk, as well. There may be times when a person who is being quiet will be asked his or her thoughts, and there may be times when a person who is talking may be asked to give others a chance to share.

e. Absences and Tardiness: For the group process to work, it is important that each group member be here on time. The flow of the group can be easily disrupted if a member comes in late or is not present each session. Also, due to the nature of this group, each session builds on the previous one, so missing one session makes it hard for the next session to be effective. If you are going to miss or be late, it is important that you let the group leader know in advance, so adjustments can be made. If a member misses more than **TWO** sessions, he/she will be asked to not attend the group anymore.

Check In Process:

Okay, we are going to do the round robin process again, and I would like for you to recall another group member's name. As this is your group, after you state another group member's name, I would also like for you to state one thing that you personally need from the others in the group for you to feel safe and or respected.
<After this is completed, ask if there are any other rules that should be added.>

Cognitive Distortion Discussion:

Cognitive distortions or as they are sometimes called thinking traps are just that traps our positive thought fall into that lead to us believing things that aren't true. These ways of thinking are based on our experiences in life, and they create negative patterns of thinking, they are based in the negative experiences of the past, and just as we predict the experiences of the future based on the past cognitive distortions lead to a constant prediction of what an experience in the present means. Interestingly, while present experiences can only be viewed based on what we have experienced, the thoughts themselves tend to distort current experiences and roadblock us from seeing current things how they really are.

There are a lot of different cognitive distortions, and listed on the worksheet are only a few of these, but what they all have in common is the fact that they change way we look at life, and it is not until we learn to identify which distortions are represent we can find a healthy way to look at those same things. healthy thoughts about an experience. The thing with cognitive distortion is that just as when we look through a bottle or a warped piece of glass, cognitive distortions make people, places, things, and events look different than they should; distorted. Most people find that they tend to view thigs through the same distortions or a combination of distortions over and over.

Overgeneralization is one type of cognitive distortion that people often will see as a present in their life and is perhaps the easiest to identify as a distorted way of thinking once the person is able to take a step back and look at an event and the statement or thought made from a logical stance. Overgeneralization is when on thinks statements which contain "always" or "never" as part of them: "She always says this." "I always fail at that." "Every time this happens, this is how my day goes." "Every guy/girl cheats." This is an example of an overgeneralization. Does every guy or girl cheat? No, there are billions of people on the planet earth, and every person doesn't cheat. Every girl or guy you have dated may have cheated on you, but you haven't dated every person, so logically it is clear that this is a distortion based on personal experiences, and thus it is those experiences which have created a way of thinking that creates a reason for why that has happened. This distortion, though, poisons healthy thought, and in turn, when you enter a relationship with these thoughts, you will assume no matter who that person is, no matter the situation, no matter what happens, eventually that person will cheat.

There are a number of other distortions, and each one has a way of poisoning healthy thoughts and overshadowing present and future experiences in a negative way. These are just some of the most common. (As each cognitive distortion is explained, ask group members to give an example.)

Overgeneralization: Allowing one or two events to be taken as proof of how someone or something thinks or acts. Overgeneralizing happens when there is the belief that something always happens or never happens.

Filtering: Extracting the good or bad of an event to focus on the negative and ignore the positive or vice versa.

Magnifying: Taking a small piece of an interaction or characteristic of a person and making it larger than it truly is. Things are blown out of proportion, and a molehill is made into a mountain.

Minimizing: Deeming a large issue to be unimportant and unworthy of focus (the opposite of magnifying).

Catastrophizing: Seeing any unpleasant occurrence as the worst possible outcome. An event may not have even happened and the expectation of how terrible it was or will be is already being considered.

Black and White Thinking: Viewing something as all or nothing. It is either good or bad; there exists no in-between. When this distortion is present, there is the lack of understanding that most times people, places, things, and events are made up of many aspects - both good and bad, right and wrong.

Blaming: Accusing another person completely for negative events occurring. Rather than accepting we did something to impact an event, our faults, failures, and other negative aspects are believed to be someone else's fault.

Personalization: Placing all the blame of something on oneself as if one had the ability to control the event entirely (opposite of blaming).

Emotional Reasoning: Removing logical aspects and focusing solely on the emotional; as a result, the person's emotions are taken as fact. An example would be "If I am scared, then there is real danger."

Mindreading: Believing one knows exactly what another person is thinking. It is mindreading that causes us to believe we know why another person did what he or she did.

Fortunetelling: Believing one knows what is going to happen before it happens. This distortion often leads the person to act in a manner which in turn creates a negative outcome.

Worksheet Review:

1. I would like each of you to tell the group a distorted thought that you have had. When the member shares this, I would like for the group to identify what distortion is present in the statement which is shared.

2. After the cognitive distortion has been identified and discussed by group members, please share why this is distorted thought; that is to say, please explain the factual aspects of the thought as well as the exceptions to the stated thought.

3. Now that the exceptions have been identified that prove this thought to be a cognitive distortion, what it the factual statement?

4. If at the time each of you had not been influenced by a cognitive distortion, but had the non-distorted factual thought, how do you think events would have turned out differently?

The ABC's of CBT

SESSION 2:

Instructions to Group Leaders:

This session is designed to teach participants Cognitive Behavioral Theory and create an understanding of the way in which a person's beliefs about an event, in turn, creates the reaction to the event.

Suggested Remarks:

Check In Process:

Last session we used the check in process to get to know each other and set up the group rules and expectations. This time, in addition to your name and the last time you drank or used, I would like you to state another group member's name and one thing that member needed to feel safe.

CBT and Patterns of Thinking:

Last week we talked about the way that cognitive distortions or thinking traps can lead to flawed thinking This week we will talk about how we change patterns of thoughts and actions. The ABC model was created to describe the way in which people react in response to an event. By understanding how we react to things, we can begin to change our reactions and how we allow events and people to impact our view of ourselves.

ABC is an acronym for the different pieces of the process. A is the Activating event: this is what happens; this is the item that starts the train of thought. It is the traffic jam, the spilled drink, the thing someone says to us. B stands for our Belief about the event: that person doesn't like me; I am always getting stuck in traffic; I can never do anything right; the world is against me. Many people explain this as the emotions and thoughts we have about what happens and combined that creates our beliefs. C is the Consequences of our thoughts and can be thought of in a few different ways. Our consequences are all of the after effects of what we believe about an event, our reaction, and the outcome.

So many people look at the event, and then they blame the event; that is the first mistake. We try to control all these things; we try to assume somehow we can change the things out of our control and change other people. The event is something that is completely out of our control- slow traffic/other people's actions - you can cuss them out all you want, but you can never control the event. Nature and others' actions are not something we will ever be able to control. We must realize this and remember that we can't control what will happen no matter what we want to happen

The next mistake that is often made is getting upset about C, our consequences of our reactions to the event. We focus on that, and we think we are wrong or bad, and that it is the reaction we need to change, but C can't be changed, not directly at least. Our reactions are the natural outcome of our beliefs and emotions created by the event that occurs.

B: B is that magical item we can control; B is that item we have the ability to directly change. Our emotions and beliefs about events are where change happens, we need to focus on and work on this item. When we make a change to B, and we feel and believe differently, C, the consequences, will naturally change as a result of the change to B.

Now expanding on ABC, there is also D and E. D and E are the creation and result of change. What D stands for is Disputing irrational beliefs, basically the process of saying "that's not true.". E is the Effective new belief that is created by the process of disputing the irrational beliefs.

When you look at this process, the important work happens at D. This is the point when we look at the facts and evidence that dispute the other beliefs to see what the real reason for the meaning behind the event. Most of the beliefs we have about events that occur and the things that others do to us are irrational. Many times, people say or do something without thinking, by mistake, or simply because they don't know better. This is an irrational belief. Even the beliefs about events that massively impact our lives are many times irrational, if we truly look at them; they have little or nothing to do with us. Traffic and a sudden storm have nothing to do with us. They will happen no matter if we were there or not, or they are something that we did by mistake, like spilling a drink. No matter what we did, we can't change them once they have happened.

The way others treat us has little to do with us and more to do with the other person. People will treat us poorly because of how they feel about themselves. It is simple psychology that people who feel like they aren't worthy often treat others like they aren't worthy. And let's say that isn't the case. Let's say that the person does something simply because he/she is mean or a jerk. Why should we care what that person thinks? Why should we care what that person says or does to us? Why should we allow it to make us feel or believe differently about ourselves?

So, when we look at the facts about the event, when we remove the emotional and look at the logical, we better understand the situation, and as a result, we naturally will create a new effective belief that is based on rational thought as well as the understanding of how our emotions impacted our belief about the situation.

Once we have disputed our beliefs about the events and we have created an effective new belief, we create F. F is the Fitting consequences; the way we react to the activating event fits the event and is not based upon irrational beliefs or emotional thought. F is an appropriate reaction to the given situation and is a healthier outcome. Just as Consequences (C) are a natural response to our Beliefs (B) and the Activating event (A), the Fitting consequences (F) are a natural result of the new Effective beliefs (E).

Now here is the thing about this process that trips people up. This change isn't instant. It is a process; it is growth, and true growth is slow. First what happens is you go through A, B, and C then later catch yourself and realize where the mistake was. Then you will slowly realize this sooner and sooner. Then what happens is you will react and almost instantly catch yourself. A little while later, you will catch yourself after the fact when you haven't reacted, and that is change. Eventually, the process is so natural that you rarely think of the change. That isn't to say it isn't a continual process because anything that can be learned can be unlearned. It is to say that by being aware when you begin to backslide you can rework the process and reinforce the change.

Worksheet Review:

Each of you completed the worksheet that examined the patterns of thoughts and challenged those patterns and I would like to see what discoveries each of you made.

1. I would like to use an open discussion approach and work through the worksheet together.

2. Who would like to share the ABC from his or her sheet? (Allow one member to discuss the ABC and his/her thoughts.)

3. Given what was just shared, what are others' thoughts on the topic? How many of you have been in a similar situation, and how did you react?

4. What would dispute the belief and emotion attached to this event, and what would be the new belief once it has been disputed?

Creating Flowing Change

SESSION 3:

Instructions to Group Leaders:

This session is designed to teach about the use of dialectical thinking. Dialectical thinking will allow participants to learn to step back and see the logical side of situations, as well as the emotional.

Suggested Remarks:

Check In Process:

As you introduce yourself and say what brought you here and the last time you drank or used, I would also like for you to share one thing that your addiction has cost you.

Dialectical Thinking:

Last session discussed the ABCDEF concept and the ways that we must change our beliefs about an event to change our reaction and the consequences related to the event. This session takes a deeper look into the process and the way which not only the process works, but how change is created. Flowcharts are used in computer programming, business, and engineering to show the process at work in a given situation step by step. Our thinking and reactions are also a process and for that reason, we can break it down step by step to understand how to effectively create change in our thinking and actions.

START – is our baseline, our worldview/lens of seeing the world. Our worldview is created by our previous interactions, our emotions, and our beliefs about the world around us and ourselves. Since our worldview can cloud our thinking, this program is designed to help with that issue and lead to change.

As discussed in the ABCDEF session, the event is something that has happened that is out of our control. The process starts with the next step in this flow chart -emotional based thought. Emotional based thought is based on our internal self-talk, the things that have happened throughout our life or the day. It is emotional not logical, and therefore, in many ways it is flawed.

Based upon emotional thinking, we form our belief about the event and we give it meaning. This meaning we then accept as fact. The belief, based on our own emotional state, contains numerous assumptions that we take as facts. When we accept assumptions, we tell ourselves we know things we do not know and allow ourselves to lean on a belief that is faulty.

Just as in ABC, our beliefs create a reaction that is based on the meaning we have given the event, through emotional thinking. This reaction is the natural progression of the process.

Out of our reaction comes the consequences; the emotional outcome is the end of the process. This is also what contributes to the creation of our worldview and, therefore, has an impact on events that follow. The emotional outcome encompasses a number of things, and can include others and the impact of our consequences on them as well. The emotional outcome is related to the individual who must deal with the repercussions of his or her own actions, but also applies to the emotional outcome for those around him or her. The consequences and emotion based outcome can be hurt feelings, physical harm, and the other things outside of our control, such as a child dealing with the loss of a parent's job.

Now that we understand all of the pieces of the first possible route from event to outcome, we look at PAUSE. Pausing is a learned skill in the process that has the ability to change every subsequent step in the process. Emotional thought will still happen, but the pause allows us to also consider the logical thought, not the emotional alone. The pause can happen at two points; it can happen after the emotional thoughts, or it can happen after those emotional thoughts have created meaning.

When we have chosen to pause, we begin down the rational or logical path. The first step in the secondary path is logic based thoughts. This means considering facts and looking at other possible reasons or causes for the activating event. Considering not only the emotional, but also the logical, is called dialectical thinking. When done correctly, it gives someone a more realistic and clear understanding of the activating event. It is at this point that we are giving dialectical thought based meaning to an event and not allowing our emotions to cause us to believe an event is something that isn't entirely true.

Just as the use of logical thought changes the belief we have about an event, it also changes our reaction to the event. That is not to say that what we initially think is always incorrect or that the reaction or outcome will always change. However, when we use dialectical thinking, most often the reaction will change, and as such, so too will the outcome. When we pause and use the dialectical path, the outcome, more often, is appropriate to the situation. This doesn't mean that there are never consequences as a result. After all, every person goes though the same processes, but it is to say that the way we react has consequences which are appropriate to the situation.

Worksheet Review:

1. Today I would like to do the review a little differently. I would like each of you to write down one situation/event, the emotional based thoughts, the meaning, and the outcome.

2. [Group leader should collect these writings, shuffle them, and pass them out to different members.]

3. As we review, I would like each of you to read the slip you have been handed and think about the logic based thought that could be connected to the event, share that logic based thought, and

discuss the way the meaning and the outcome would change based on that thought and meaning.

Family Patterns of Addiction and the Stages of Change

SESSION 4:

Instructions to Group Leaders:

This session is designed to teach group participants about the patterns of addiction within families and how genetics and environment both contribute to these patterns. This session with also designed to teach group members about the stages of change and understand the process of recovery. Each stage will be explained, and group members should be able to identify their own progress and current stage.

Suggested Remarks:

Check In Process:

This session I would like to use the check in process to talk about what you have learned so far. As you check in with your name and date of last use, I would also like for you to say one thing that you have learned so far or what has had the most impact on you.

Family Patterns:

Addiction often runs through families and the substance of choice may vary within a family, but the patterns can be contributed to many aspects. The two main contributors, genetics and environment, can both contribute to patterns of addiction in families.

Research presented to Congress in April of 2008 showed that "at least half of a person's susceptibility to drug addiction can be linked to genetic factors" (APA). On a basic cellular level, each person has material that came from their mother and father, which in turn means they also have parts of them which came from their mom's parents and their dad's parents, and so on back up the family tree. Because our genes determine the makeup of who we are on a physical level this means that the physical aspect of addiction can be seen when looking across the generations of a family. One or both of you parents may have or have had an addiction issue, smoking, alcohol, other drugs, or neither of them may have, but often if a person has an addiction issue they will find blood related family who also has addiction issues, grandparents, an aunt or uncle, a sibling and if there exists a pattern within the family this may mean that you are more likely to develop an addiction issue.

Environment is the second major factor in patterns of addiction within families; what you are exposed to within the family where you were raised. Unlike the genetic factor which related only to birth families, environment can be a factor for either biological or non-biological families and create a pattern of addiction for non-blood related family members. When we look at environment we are looking at what parents, grandparents, and other caregivers were seen doing or what the environment where a person was raised was like. There are two pieces to environment as family patterns of addiction.

If as a child, you watch your father smoke or drink every night when he gets home as a way to relax the chance that you will use this same way to distress is increased. If your mother was addicted to drugs and you watched as she used drugs over and over you are more likely to try drugs as a result. The National Center of Addiction and Substance Abuse at Columbia University found that "teens who have seen their parent(s) drunk are more than twice as likely to get drunk in a typical month, and three times likelier to use marijuana and smoke cigarettes." Parents and family members who use drugs, alcohol, or smoke also contribute to the increased likelihood of a teen trying these substances because they often have easier access to substances.

In addition to watching other people use substances, another environmental factor which increases the chance a person will try substances and become addicted is what the environment in the home is like. Having parents or caregivers who are regularly in conflict or a home where frequent conflict or aggressive behaviors exist. Having at least one parent who is depressed or has other psychological issues can lead to an increased chance of family patterns of addiction, or that person having addiction related issues. These factors along with experiencing neglect all elevate the chance that an addiction issue can develop, these can also be signs that a hidden addiction already exists since all of these items are more likely to happen when one of the parents, or both are addicted to alcohol or drugs.

Now while family patterns of addiction occur and your genetics and environment can determine the likelihood of if you will may have a problem with addiction each of us make a conscious choice to try and continue use of substances. There may be a psychological and/or physical connection to your use or addiction you hold the power to change that cycle as it may currently exist.

Stages of Change in Recovery:

It is generally accepted that there are six stages of recovery; everyone who is creating change (anyone in recovery) will go through the stages in order, even if he or she is not aware of going through the stages. Understanding what stage you are at in the recovery and change process is important as it serves in some ways as a protective and motivating force.

<u>Pre-contemplation</u>: This is a stage that precedes change. During the pre-contemplation phase, a person may realize there are negative outcomes to his or her behavior, but doesn't believe the behavior is problematic, so there is no need to change. At this stage alcoholics or addicts often believe that those around them are the ones with a problem.

<u>Contemplation</u>: This is the stage where change truly begins. During the contemplation phase, a person begins to question if he or she has a problem and needs to make changes. At this stage there is

commonly a large amount of back and forth between believing help and change is needed and the rejection of this idea.

Preparation: This stage is the point when a person begins to prepare to take action. During the preparation phase, an individual has accepted responsibility for his or her actions and understands that change needs to occur. It is at this point one begins to gather information or seek referrals for help. A person may also set a timeline for his or her treatment.

Action: This is the stage where the work is done. It is during the action phase that individuals enter into treatment, be it AA, residential programs, or outpatient therapy. At this stage there is an emotional, mental, and spiritual engagement in the change process. New skills and understanding are gained and put into use to create a shift in addiction-related behavior and create sobriety and recovery.

Maintenance: This is the stage where a person has made adjustments to his or her behavior and patterns of thinking, thus gaining an understanding of self and actions. These skills have become a part of one's behavior, and they are utilized to create a new routine. It is during the maintenance phase that most people leave residential treatment and return to their everyday lives.

Relapse: This is a return to substance use, and it often occurs as a part of recovery. Unlike the other stages, relapse can happen at any point during the process. It can happen during preparation, action, and maintenance. No matter where relapse occurs, an individual return back to pre-contemplation, but most generally once the substances are out of a person's system, he or she quickly returns to the action stage and subsequently to maintenance with additional understanding resulting from relapse.

Worksheet Review:

1. First each of you has a choice to either share or not to share any family patterns of addiction you may know to exist or believe may exist, but you do not have to.

2. I would like for each of you to share what stage of the change process you feel you are currently in.

3. Why did you choose preparation, action, or maintenance?
[Correct members if they choose the wrong stage and explain differences.]

4. What does each of you need to move along to the next stage? What is preventing your progress? Are there people who can assist you with this progress?

The Recovery Battle

SESSION 5:

Instructions to Group Leaders:

This session is designed to aid group members with understanding those things which can stand in the way of their recovery, the items and people who may attack and tear down the defenses against relapse, and the people and things which can help protect and defend recovery and sobriety.

Suggested Remarks:

Check In Process:

Today I would like each of you to introduce yourself, and a mountain and a valley from your week (one positive thing and one negative thing).

The Battle for Recovery:

Understanding what can impact continued recovery and lead to relapse is a highly important piece of protecting your recovery. Knowing the pitfalls that may occur and the negative events, people, and places that have a high chance of leading to relapse can help prevent the impact of those items.

Most people are able to identify the dragons, the big triggers that will have a huge impact on them and the highest likelihood of putting them in a position where they may use drugs or alcohol. These items are the places that you spend time: friends' houses, parties, sporting events, these places can be directly tied to drinking and the use of other substances. Another example may be watching sports or large family gatherings. Again, these events may be connected to drinking and substance use in celebration or as a way of coping with the occasions.

Often connected to these places are people who have a strong ability to weaken a person's recovery and identifying these people helps to protect your recovery by avoidance and awareness. Obviously, your drug dealer isn't the ideal person to spend time with when you are in recovery, but neither are the friends who you spent large amounts of time with where drinking or drug use occurred, and even family and partners who use and abuse substances and who are unwilling to stop the use around you can be destructive. Early in recovery it is important to avoid these people, sometimes permanently, or could be temporary.

It is also important to know what the dragon's fire is; the methods that they use to weaken your recovery. It is important to know what weakens your recovery because long-term recovery is not about avoidance, but about awareness and acceptance of addiction. You need to identify limits and know where defense is needed.

While large attackers and threats to your recovery are like dragons and easy to identify, it is also important to identify the lesser threats to sustained recovery. Who or what are the archers in your life, and what are the slings and arrows they will use to attack you? These people and things are often far harder to identify, and the reason for this is they may be less overt in their attempts to influence you, or they may simply be the stressors and emotions that make you desire to use. Work could be an archer and boredom be the arrow, or a friend who drinks or uses drugs may never ask you to join them, but may make references to use that can cause a desire to drink and use substances.

The benefit of this recovery battle is that you are not in the battle unarmed and you are not alone. What is your shield that protects you? Is it your faith? Is it your goals? Is it your awareness? Whatever this is, it is important to continue to develop it. Your shield is your coping skills and the things you have learned in treatment. These items are your protection, and just as a knight holds tight to his shield, make sure you hold tight to yours, as well.

Lastly, but just as important, is identifying those people who will stand with you and protect your recovery. Only you can choose recovery, and only your actions determine if relapse occurs, but others are still there to support and reinforce your recovery. Alcoholic Anonymous or Narcotics Anonymous and other support groups are key to maintaining recovery for many, but for others it may be faith or some other group. If these organizations are part of the shield, the individuals like sponsors, ministers, and family members are your comrades and the ones who help hold you up and maintain recovery when you feel weak, but they are unable to hold the shield for you. They are unable to maintain your recovery; that is a choice that must be made by you alone.

Worksheet Review:

1. Today's worksheet was a little more fun in nature, but the reality is that sobriety and recovery are battles which each person either wins or loses. For some the big dragon is the toughest fight, but for others, it is the constant barrage of arrows.

2. What is the big attacker of your sobriety, and what are the smaller attackers? Which is the tougher fight? Why?

3. What are the people and things that help protect you and your recovery? What if those items were to suddenly disappear? How would you continue to protect your recovery?

Use Recall Protection

SESSION 6:

Instructions to Group Leaders:

This session is designed to help group members prevent relapse through gaining a better understanding of what has led to past desires to drink and/or use substances as well as understanding of the cues and self-talk that has led to use.

Suggested Remarks:

Check In Process:

To start, I would like each of you to introduce yourself, and then tell the group what stage of the recovery process you are in currently. I also would like you to answer how you are feeling, but only use mad, glad, sad, or afraid. [See check in process in beginning of manual]

Prevention and Use Recall:

The greatest tool in preventing substance use and relapse, related to addiction or not, is to understand what you thought and what you felt when you chose to drink or use substances in the past. Oftentimes when assessing past activities, one will find that people, places, and events share common emotional reactions that lead to similar internal self-talk. These emotions and self-talk can lead to mental, physical, and behavioral cues, all of which play off one another to create a perfect storm that has the potential to lead to relapse.

Vignette:

> *You are texting with your girlfriend or boyfriend and they are angry. The two of you begin to argue. As the argument progresses, you start to feel angry, sad, and hurt by the things that are being said. In the heat of the argument, you block his or her number and you go jump in your car and take off. As you are driving, you begin to tell yourself how worthless you are, how you deserve better, or how you are a loser for picking someone like him or her. You keep thinking how you want to get high. You remind yourself how your friend always has something to smoke. You find yourself heading to that friend's house, even though you were just aimlessly driving. You also are wrenching the steering wheel as you are driving. You feel flush and hot inside, and you are almost panting because you are so angry.*

(As you go through the discussion, have group members identify the different items in the above example for each section.)

Psychologically, substance abuse relapse and self-medicating tend to connect to the same thought patterns over and over as it reoccurs. It is by identifying these patterns that a person is able to stop the cascading items that lead to substance and to prevent relapse in the future.

As you work through this examination of past use, the first thing that each person should do is to look at the past times when drinking or substance abuse occurred and look at the situations surrounding those instances. This is a two-part examination for the fact that there are situations when a person tends to use and there are situations that can precede a person relapsing or using. The first part of this examination is to look at the situations when you drink or use drugs: are these sporting events, parties, or specific people? Even if it is family and friends that lead you to drink in celebration, these situations should be avoided early on in recovery because these are some of the hardest and weakest times for people. Over time, as a person's recovery strengthens and becomes a part of him or her, these events can be added back in, but early in recovery. The second part of examining situations when you use, is to look at the triggers that cause you to want to drink or use substances. These are not the times when you use alcohol or another substance, but the interactions that happen before and lead to your desire to use. This can be any number of things, but often they are stressful or highly emotional situations where a person feels the best way to relieve the emotional charge is to use alcohol or other drugs to self-medicate. One of the most common situations which leads to use and relapse are interpersonal and romantic relationships such as close friends, family, and romantic partners. Relationship interactions are some of the most emotionally charged interactions that one encounters, and due to the fact substance use is tied very closely with emotions, this means some relationships have a high likelihood of creating situations where relapse can occur. When identifying these type of situations, you are looking at the triggers; interactions, and emotions, and responses after which you have the strongest desire to use, such as dramatic interactions like fights with a significant other, or a funeral.

The next step in this proactive recall exercise is to look at the feelings which precede a desire to use or caused past relapse situations. As stated earlier, there tends to be a pattern in each individual's use as far as emotions are concerned. Even opposing emotions that can cause a desire to use in the same individual; love and anger, arrogance and disappointment, joy and sorrow. When you are assessing these emotions and feelings that lead to a desire to use or caused past substance use, there is the need to be brutally honest with yourself about what you were feeling. What you should not do is place a judgment of good or bad on the emotion. This process is not about judging yourself for what you feel; it is about understanding the emotions inside that can hinder your recovery and lead to relapse.

Self-talk is the internal message that each of us carries around within ourselves, and those messages can impact your recovery. Identify the little things you tell yourself - the thoughts and the messages that give you a reason or an excuse to drink. These can be different things, including blaming others, telling yourself you deserve it, or telling yourself you are a loser. All of these messages are self-talk that may make a person want to drink or use substances, and creates habits. These habits create urges and, as such, are all items of concern for relapse.

Cues can be mental, physical, or behavioral, but they are all signals of a desire to use substances and can be warning signs that help protect recovery and prevent relapse.

Mental Cues

Mental cues are connected to our self-talk. They are related to the way we think about substance use. Mental cues can be widespread in nature, ranging from what you believe about yourself or the world to thinking that drinking or drug use is the answer to a problem. Preceding relapse, often there is the glamorizing or euphoric remembrance of the times when a person drank or used drugs. Fantasizing is an often-occurring mental cue that, if left unchecked, commonly leads to relapse.

Physical Cues

Physical cues are indicators of an urge or craving to use based on internal and autonomic reactions; things that which happen without our awareness or control. Common cues attached to urges and a desire to use are things like a change in breathing, increased heart rate, feeling flush or cool. Cues are something that are very individual experiences. While two people may have shared cues, rarely will they share all of the same cues connected to every situation. For some people, when they are angry their ears turn red, but for others, breathing may increase, and still others may have some sort of an eye twitch. All of these are physical cues (another thing to remember is that a physical cue mean something different for each person, even if it looks the same. A good example of this is someone's face turning red. Is it the result of anger, embarrassment, or amusement? Recognizing your physical cues can help an individual also recognize precursors to potential relapse.

Behavioral Cues

Behavioral cues are often confused with physical cues but are exactly what they sound like, how you act. A physical cue is something that will happen on its own – breathing, heartbeat, eye twitch. Conversely, behavioral cues are learned behaviors that are connected to emotions. Pacing, gritting your teeth, wrenching your hands, and talking to yourself are all behavioral cues. Like all the other cues listed above, behavioral cues are things that happen without conscious thought, yet they are activities that we can be aware of and stop.

Worksheet Review:

1. What I would like us to do is go around and discuss the situations, people, places, things, and events which have created a desire to use in the past. While there is the need to be respectful as each person shares, I would like others to share if this has been a difficult situation for you, as well.

2. Now that the exterior components have been discussed, I would like to talk about the emotions which have led to continued use or past relapse. While the events, places, and situations may be different what is commonly shared are emotions. *I may not have been through what you've been through, but I have felt what you felt, and thought what you thought.*

Responsive vs. Reactive

SESSION 7:

Instructions to Group Leaders:

This session is designed to assist group members in further understanding the impact emotions have on the way in which a person reacts. A clear understanding of responsive and reactive behaviors will be discussed to aid in the evaluation of actions and reactions. It is designed to help each person to better understand his/her own vulnerabilities and internal messages. Most importantly, it is about how trigger events impact us.

Suggested Remarks:

Check In Process:

For check in I would like each of you to answer the standard questions: name, last date of use, and what stage of recovery you are in and we will do mountains and valleys.

Responsive versus Reactive:

When discussing responsive versus reactive, the analogy of stairs is used because it is a fitting example that most people can visualize and apply more easily to their own experiences. To help with visualization, think back to your childhood and picture Bugs Bunny, Tom and Jerry, or another cartoon. The character is walking along and steps on a roller skate, a banana peel, or, as in the worksheet, the character trips over a rock. With any cartoon there are only two common outcomes, depending often on if the character is the hero or villain. The villain will hit this obstacle and will stumble around or go sliding off and end up tumbling head over heel down a flight of dark stairs. The heroes turn this obstacle into some type of superpower, however. They surf or ski their way to a wondrous outcome, getting where they wanted to go that much quicker, or they trip over the rock, and it turns into some great flip with a flawless dismount that makes their climb a simple task. When talking about the hero or villain, the important thing to keep in mind is the fact they are one in the same. They are both inside each of us, and it is our internal message we allow to influence our thinking that, in turn, leads to the outcome.

We want to look at each step in this process. What is being sought is not just an understanding of how our beliefs impact the outcomes, but it is looking deeper to understand our internal messages. Each person carries through life different internal messages that are both reinforced by and create vulnerabilities and our beliefs about events. Internal messages are those things that we tell ourselves.

Some pieces of these messages are easy to identify; you make a mistake, and you tell yourself "I am so stupid." Someone dumps you, and you say "no one will ever love me." Other pieces of these messages are much deeper. Where did they come from? How are they reinforced? How do they impact my life? These questions are what this exercise is designed to answer, and to do so, the worksheet is designed to be worked backwards. Just like the cartoon, hit rewind and watch the antagonist tumble up the stairs.

Start with the worst outcome or consequence of a recent drinking or drug use event. What was the end result? It should be noted while this is an emotional exercise, this isn't about judging yourself. It is about understanding why you judge yourself the way you do. So, what was the basement floor, the negative end result of the last use? Was it a bad grade, a breakup, or friend? A car wreck or a hole punched in the wall and things broken? Now work backwards each step. What actions led to that - your actions, not other people's actions. With each step up, you should also be thinking about what self-talk you were telling yourself, and how with each preceding step the self-talk not only worsened the next step, but also intensified the self-talk.

Now work yourself back to the trigger event. What was that? Ask yourself something very key. Why did it lead to the reaction that it did? This reason is tied to your internal message, and each time a trigger led to use, it reinforced that same train of thought. If you walk through life believing you are a failure or not good enough, and then if I fail a test my reaction will be one of destructive behavior, going and having a drink, going and buying drugs, telling someone we love they are worthless, throwing something and breaking it. Similarly, if you walk through life believing you are superior to everyone and you fail a test, the same results can play out. You are fail a test. You think you deserve better and the next test you will ace, so you go and drink or use. You go home and get in a fight over a bad grade and then getting high or drunk. You tear down family members or friends to remind them that they are beneath you, and on and on. Here is the interesting thing. Most times, for these two types of people, the deepest internal message is the exact same one, but there is a cover message that tries to fight the negative message with a positive one.

Everyone carries an internal message, and it comes from a young age. It does not change; it is a part of each person's personality. What is important is the understanding of what the internal message is and what events will serve to reinforce it as well as the way it has impacted past events. This understanding can completely shift the outcome of future events.

We hit rewind, and we watched Tom bounce up the basement stairs, flip onto the skate, and hop off when we rewound the negative events. Now play these events forward with the understanding of your internal message. When the event happens, what happens if your internal message doesn't lead to substance use? Does getting fired still lead to drinking if you know your self-talk is your insecurities and vulnerabilities pushing to remind you how worthless you are, and, in turn, create an excuse or reason to relapse? When you don't relapse, do you go home and yell at your parents, or do you talk to them about sadness or hurt? Do you call your parents names, or do you say "I love you"? Do you break things, or do you talk about how you will work together and study harder? Let your event play out, but imagine that your self-talk was positive not negative. When you are impacted by your vulnerabilities, remind yourself of the logical side and that it was only your internal message.

Do this with a number of events - any number of times that you used, and even times that you didn't, and keep a list of what that first thought was when you experienced the trigger event. The more that you walk yourself through events, the better you will understand the nature of your internal message. Through this understanding of your own internal message, you can change the outcomes and strengthen your self-esteem and recovery.

Homework Review:

1. Show of hands: How many of you feel like you were already aware of your reacting/responding habits? Show of hands again: How many of you were surprised by this?
2. For those who were surprised, I would like you to share what surprised you in the process of completing this exercise. Also, I would like you to share how you think you will learn to function in a more responsive way if you were reactive.
3. For those who already understood they were reactive, not responsive, the question I want you to think about and to answer when it is your turn is this: If you are aware you are reactive, what have you begun doing to help shift that pattern, and if nothing, why?

The Three Whos of Me

SESSION 8:

Suggested Remarks:

Check In Process:

This week for part of check in I would like you think about who you are, as we go around the circle I would like each of you to share something that you think defines who you are that others may not know.

The Three Whos:

Who am I? This is a question all people ask at one time or another. Defining who we are is a difficult thing because we tend to look for one idea, one perfect picture of who we are. The reality is that each of us has many sides to us, many roles we fill, many things we feel and think. They may be contradictions to each other, but who we are is important to discover, because it tells us who we are not, and *we can or want to be*.

We all have different sides based on who we are around or what the setting is. How you act at home most likely is different than how you act when you are at work or school. How you interact and what you say to your parents or other family members is most likely different than how you interact with your friends. All of these are natural, and in fact, even if they are different they are still the true you. However, there are also things we do, ways we act, things we say, which are masks that we put on to play a part. This can be due to a number of factors; the most common is peer pressure, but there is also family pressure and self-talk that can impact how we act and why we wear masks.

According to an online search. "Peer-pressure is the direct influence on people by peers, or the effect on an individual who gets encouraged to follow their peers by changing their attitudes, values or behaviors to conform to those of the influencing group or individual." Peer-pressure can be direct or indirect, it can be someone directly saying you should drink or simply being in a setting where all of your friends are drinking. The desire to fit in with friends is one of the strongest influences on adolescents' and teens' thoughts and behaviors and it can create a lot of masks as a result. The expectation of family to conform to their desired picture of who you are can cause us to wear masks as well. If you are raised in a very conservative or religious home and you are gay you may create a mask to fit the beliefs of your family.

Realizing that there are many different parts to who you are and who you pretend to be is an important part of making better choices. I may be a kind person, but my friends pick on someone else and to fit in I make jokes or pretend to laugh about that. I may not want to drink or use drugs, but the people I hang out with may use drugs and to fit in I use. Some of you are probably sitting in this room for that very reason.

Today's exercise is designed to help you think about the different roles you play and realize who the real you is versus who you pretend to be.

On the worksheet below write the words that you believe describe you in the different areas of your life. While the sheet is divided into three sections to focus on the "real me", the "masks I wear", and "who I want to be", you can divide these sections more if you desire as friend section, family section, emotion sections, setting sections, however you like. You may also choose to draw items you associate with these areas.

As part of this project I would like you to use the supplies to either draw, glue, or write in each section. How you divide the sections and answer the three questions are up to you, but all three need to be included as part of the project.

The first section is "who are you", who is the real you in whatever situation, with friends, with family, at school. You will most likely find common themes such as funny, caring, the silly one. The more you think about who you are in different situations you will find who the real you is.

Who do you pretend to be? Look at the masks you wear and try to understand the things that you do to make others believe you fit in. These things will generally be things that you are uncomfortable with doing, but not always. Some of the masks we wear we have worn so long we don't know that we are pretending anymore.

The third piece is "who you want to be" which may be connected to masks, it may be who you would like to be in the future as far as success. Who you want to be can be connected to the changes you would like to make in your life, not just what future job would you like, what kind of car you want to drive. It is connected to who you want to be as a person and how you want to feel about yourself in the future.

You should write in each section your thoughts and/or lists of what you think about these three sections of your life. You should also use the other items provided to either draw depictions or glue pictures of those things you like, that represents those three sections, and what you want to be true about you. You can divide the paper however you wish to separate the three parts. If you have a difficult time starting, try drawing a shape that you feel represents you and dividing that in thirds or a shape you feel represents each question.

Poster Project:

Give group participants 30-45 minutes to work on their posters. As work on them allow free conversation between group participants as a matter of healthy and appropriate communication and interaction. If needed use prompting questions to illicit discussion.

- What is your dream job?
- What do you like to do in your spare time?
- What is something that you once enjoyed that you stopped doing when you began using?
- If you could be anything in the world what would it be and why?

Poster Review:

Once the project is finished asked for volunteers to share their poster.

Ask each individual to discuss why drawings, quotes, or pictures were added to a specific section. Ensure you expand on items which stand out or are clinically significant. Ask question as needed to engage quieter group members or who have added an image which seems worthy of discussion or out of place. A youth may add a picture of a Pokémon or another video game or cartoon character to the "who I want to be" section, this may represent they want to be in animation, it may represent a desire to program or be a professional gamer, these are areas to encourage a youth for growth. This same picture may simply be added and the youth states "I don't plan to work and just play video games all day" this would be an area to question the benefit and/or reality of this idea.

Event Assessments

SESSION 9:

Instructions to Group Leaders:

This session is designed to help group participants learn to assess events and understand the manner in which logical thought, emotional thought, and perceptions combine to create the reality each person experiences.

Suggested Remarks:

Check In Process:

Please introduce yourself, state your last date of use, and what stage you are currently in, and your mountains and valleys from this week.

Learning to Assess Events:

The way we view an event is rarely the full picture. We must evaluate an event before determining the truth. Evaluating an event from different perspectives allows us to understand ourselves better as well; what makes us happy, what triggers cravings and use.

What we are looking for in this whole process is to understand how all of the perspectives of the process create the reality in which we live. Reality can best be viewed as the place where an event, the facts of the event, and our vulnerabilities all intersect. Additionally, within this spot is also the intersection of emotional thought, logical thought, and our perception of events.

When doing this assessment, the event or trigger is the first thing to examine. What happened that started it all? That is to say, what was the first event that led to those urges or cravings? What started you down that path: was it a break up, being late to work, getting fired, or a celebration with friends? Once we have stated the event or trigger, we then want to think about the facts of the situation, because what happened it is not always what truly happened.

Facts are a key piece in this as they help to pull us out of the emotional state in which we exist. After all, as humans, emotions impact most everything we experience, do, say, and think. So, what are the facts of the situation? Sure, facts can be unpleasant, but they remain facts regardless. The interesting thing about pulling the facts out of an event is that when we do that, we also see what our vulnerabilities and fears are. Vulnerabilities are often viewed as weaknesses, but they are better described as insecurities since once we understand them, they can be turned into strengths. Insecurities can be strengths? The answer is yes.

As stated earlier, reality is not only the place where the event, facts, and vulnerabilities intersect, but reality is created by the combination of emotional thought, logical thought, and our perceptions. First, we will address emotional thought because that is often our first response, however, emotional thought is not fact. It is not even fact based.

Perceptions are created by overlapping facts and vulnerabilities which are connected to an event or trigger. Our vulnerabilities remain within us regardless of the trigger or facts about the event. For example, view facts as clear water and vulnerabilities as dirt; when dirt is added to water, the water's clarity gets muddied. The muddy water becomes the perception of the event.

Interestingly, logical thought is not the whole truth either. Rather, it should be described as not our entire reality, but where the majority of the truth of a situation exists. Logical thought is what we strive for to avoid relapse, drinking, drug use, and all destructive behaviors. Logical thought is the last piece most people acknowledge, and while it is a part of reality, it is the piece that is seldom looked at before drinking or drug use occurs. Logical thought is found by comparing the alternative causes for a situation and considering if what we perceive as reality is based upon an emotional reaction rather than the facts of the event that occurred.

Worksheet Review:

1. I would like to know in general what each of you thought about the worksheet from last week?
2. Was there any aspect of this process that was surprising to anyone?
3. For each of you, what was the vulnerability you found was most common in your thinking? [write on white board if available]
4. How many of you can identify with the items listed on the board, even if the items aren't your most common vulnerability? How many of you have experienced those items identified by other group members?

Change Plans

SESSION 10:

Instructions to Group Leaders:

This session is designed to help members understand the process of creating a change plan. It is a discussion about the different parts that are included in a change plan and the way which creating change plan assists in promoting change.

Suggested Remarks:

Check In Process:

For check in, I would like each of you to answer the normal questions—name & last date of use. Additionally, I would like each person to say something good that has happened since the last session.

Creating a Change Plan:

Any time we are trying to create a change or grow as a person, the key is the development of a plan; a stated way to understand what growth we are looking to achieve and know how to get there. In this change plan, there are set steps which can make planning and evaluation a much easier process and help make reaching a goal or creating a change easier.

In most cases, the natural place to start the creation of a change plan is by stating what is it you want to change or achieve. Once you have identified the goal or change, it is hugely important to understand what the motivation for change is and what value is connected to that motivation. The reason motivation and values are key is when we start to falter and backslide, being reminded of the motivating factors and the values that drive the change can serve as reinforcement to continue towards the goal.

Once there is the understanding of what is motivating the change, the next step is identifying what it takes to reach the goal. If someone says he/she wants to lose 10 pounds, that is a goal. It is a definable, measureable change, but to reach that goal, there are steps along the way. A person doesn't just achieve weight loss by thinking about it. He or she works towards it step by step. The steps may be a change in diet, the creation of a workout regime, etc., which help reach that ultimate goal of losing 10 pounds. These steps need to be definable as well as measurable. "I will work out more" is too vague, "I will work out X number of hours, X number of days a week" is a defined and measurable step toward the goal. Along with defining measurable steps, it is important to also attach a timeline to these steps and the ultimate goal. This is not to say that if the set timeline passes you cannot reevaluate the completion date, but when people place a timeframe on events, it tends to push them to work towards goals, and a set date is, again, measurable.

With anything in life, there are those things which can promote change and those things which can hinder change. Identifying the people, places, and things which can help with reaching a goal will help you know what to lean on in the hard times and who can help encourage you to work towards the goal. Similarly, it is important to know who the people are and what the places and things are which will hold you back and could encourage stagnation and failure rather than promote growth. Spending time with a friend who likes to jog might be a great inspiration to lose weight and keep working towards that goal. Running with that friend past your favorite fast food place may not be the best idea.

How do you know if your plan is working or not working? This is why making steps and tasks which are measurable and have timeframes attached to them is so important; after all, it is hard to measure if you are reaching your goal if there are not well-defined milestones and markers to help identify progress. And the last step is to define what can be done if the plan isn't working. Some people want to avoid this step as they see it as an excuse to fail, but the reality is that this step helps identify what to change if the current plan isn't working before any setbacks occur.

All the steps in a change plan are fluid in nature. Start with a plan, but be open to adapting it as you go. If running isn't working to lose weight, or avoiding others isn't helping you to not drink, it is necessary to identify other items which will work and will promote change. The steps all include self-reflection and evaluation to ensure the creation of lasting change. Self-reflection also helps ensure the reason for the change is based on our own desires and values. For if it is solely based upon the desires of those around us, the change is likely to be temporary and less motivating.

Worksheet Review:

1. So each person created a change plan. Some of you may have created more than one plan because you have more than one change you want to create. I would like each person to discuss the change plan created connected to the one goal each of you has in common, like continued sobriety and recovery.

2. Instead of working through every part of the change plan for each person, let's talk about the aspects that were the hardest to answer or which were confusing for members. What were these items? [Ask group members to help each other.]

Two Letter Exercise

ORIENTATION AND GRADUATION PROJECT:

Orientation Session:

As part of the Orientation session the letter to me project should be explained as it relates to the letter which is expected prior to the first group session and the letter which will be written and read to the class at the individual's last group session.

The first of these two letters should be written before the individual is allowed to start the first group. This letter should address several items, but should not be read before the group, maybe explored by the therapist with the individual in the first individual session, but should be sealed in an envelope and kept for the individual. The letter should answer most of the following basic questions:

1. Why are you here for treatment?
2. If you could change what brought you here what would you do differently, if anything?
3. What is your thought about being in treatment?
4. What do you believe you will get out of treatment?
5. Where do you think you will be in approximately 12 weeks when you complete your treatment?
6. What do you see your overall future looking like?

After the youth completes this letter the therapist should review it with the individual and can ask the individual for clarification, but the ideas in the letter should not be challenged at this point as the youth is most likely in a pre-contemplative stage and challenging the letter will most likely be viewed as judgment and can shut down the individual and damage the development of a therapeutic relationship.

Graduation Group Session:

As part of the last session for the youth, the graduation session, every group member should be required to write a letter to him or herself related to changes which have occurred over the last 12 weeks. The letter should be written not in a report format, but in a format which is more in line with the youth writing to him or herself from before entering treatment. Addressed in this letter should be the following items:

1. What are your thoughts on what brought you to treatment?
2. If you could change anything about what brought you to treatment would you, if so, what and why?
3. What are your thoughts about the person you were before entering treatment?
4. If you could tell yourself anything about treatment what would it be?

5. What have you learned about yourself, your drug use, or other topics as a result of having been involved in treatment?
6. What is you view of the future after having been through this program?

Each individual should read their letter aloud to the other group members at the end of their final session. To ensure that there is enough time for this and goodbyes to occur ensure that you either reserve 10 minutes at the end of this group for the graduating individual or that you are able to extend the group to ensure time for the letter to be read to the group.

Relapse Prevention Planning

INDIVIDUAL SESSION:

Preventing Relapse

Having worked through this program, you have gained a greater understanding of what emotional and physical triggers have impacted how you feel about yourself and have gained an understanding of your addiction. Recovery is a daily practice, and one of the best ways to protect that recovery on a daily basis is to have a relapse prevention plan.

As you complete the relapse prevention plan below, you will find items that connect to all the aspects discussed over the course of this group. Every group, every exercise, all of your work to this point has been preparing you to go out into life and manage and protect your recovery.

1. Look at the events that led to using and that may have led to relapse previously. These are some situations which may be triggers in the future, as well.
2. Consider the emotions you felt when the event occurred, or the emotions which have led to use or relapse, regardless of the event or situation.
3. Continue to the thoughts you had, your perceptions, your reality, your self-talk.
4. List the possible negative impacts of using
5. Look at the positives of sobriety.
6. Three of the most important questions related to your continued recovery are: who can you talk to, what else can you do, and what are the emotional outcomes of continued recovery. The first two questions help remind you who your supports are. None of us are alone; yet different situations may require us to talk to different people. Remember activities that help stop thoughts of relapse or alleviate stress before the thoughts of relapse happen are supports we do for ourselves
7. The last question, *what is the emotional outcome of continued recovery*, relates to your values and motivation that led to change and a reminder of the need to protect your recovery in good times but especially in not so good times.

- **Where were you? What were you doing?**
-

- **What emotions were you feeling? How intense (1-10)?**
-

- **What were your negative thoughts?**
-

- **What are the outcomes of relapse?**
- 1.
-
- 2.
-
- 3.
-
- 4.
-
- 5.
-

- **What are the outcomes of not using?**
- 1.

2.

3.

4.

5.

- **What can you do instead of drinking/using?**
-
-

•   •
• **Who can you talk to about the situation?**   •   •   •   •
• **What is the emotional outcome of continued recovery?**   •   •   •   •

Discharge Session:

INDIVIDUAL SESSION:

Relapse Prevention Plan Review:

The final discharge session should occur as soon after completion of group program sessions. As part of this session a relapse prevention plan should be presented by the individual. This plan should have been discussed in previous individual sessions and should have evolved over the course of 12 weeks of group and individual sessions. The plan should be discussed and an understanding of the items on the plan should be assessed by the therapist. Additionally, the therapist should give feedback of possible additional items which might be of assistance to the plan if there are any that the therapist has observed or believes to be missing for the individual's Relapse Prevention Plan,

If this Relapse Prevention Plan has not been completed, then the exercise addressed in the first required individual session should be again addressed with the individual and the plan completed for a successful discharge to occur.

Letter Exercise:

As part of the discharge planning session the letter which was written prior to starting the group therapy sessions should be provided to the individual. The therapist should have the individual read the letter and give feedback about what was thought prior to treatment and what the current thoughts are about treatment and the progress which has been made. At this point it is acceptable and appropriate for the therapist to question any negative, misguided, or incorrect statements and/or thoughts which may be contained in this first letter.

Made in United States
Orlando, FL
04 November 2026

90200627R00026